THIS PAGE

INTENTIONALLY LEFT

BLANK

@2019 by Ronnie Manns. All rights reserved.

No part of this book may be reproduced, stored in a retrieval system, or transmitted by any means, electronic, mechanical, photocopying, recording, or otherwise, without written permission from the author.

First self-published by Ronnie Manns 05/02/19

ISBN-9781096668190

Printed in the United States of America

Queen Creek, AZ

This book is printed on acid free paper.

Table of Contents

PREFACE

I dedicate this to my wife Susan M. Manns and my mother Dollie J. Manns who stands with me long after all others leave. It is not often you find those who are willing to love you enough to tell you the truth in all instances holding back nothing except the cruelest way of telling you. These two earth angels have a way of telling me the worst of news in a manner that makes me glad to hear it. You can always tell those who are saying things to help and those who are saying things to hurt. I shall never fear what they may say and always look forward to what they do.

The Definition and Origination of Mental Illness

The National Alliance on Mental Illness (NAMI) defines mental illness as "a condition that affects a person's thinking, feeling or mood" but my truth says that in addition to this, mental illness is further defined as the result of a traumatic event which occurs whether you are involved in it or simply happen to witness it. These two things in combination are borne out in the latest explanations espoused by those experts who we have come to depend on and trust to know the truth about mental illnesses.

The American Psychiatric Association explains that "mental illnesses are associated with distress and/or problems functioning in social, work or family activities. Mental illnesses take many forms. Some are mild and only interfere in limited ways with daily life, such as certain phobias (abnormal fears). Other mental health conditions are so severe that a person may need care in a hospital." while the Mayo Clinic warns that "mental illness is a leading cause of disability. Untreated mental illness can cause severe emotional, behavioral and physical health problems. The effects of mental illness can be temporary or long lasting. You also can have more than one mental health disorder at the same time."

Many of the leading experts in the field of mental health agree that there are other factors which may attribute to the cause of mental illness. NAMI speaks to this by saying "a mental health condition isn't the result of one event. Research suggests multiple, linking causes. Genetics, environment and lifestyle influence whether someone develops a mental health condition. A stressful job or home life makes some people more susceptible, as do traumatic life events like being the victim of a crime. Biochemical processes and circuits and basic brain structure may play a role, too and the Mayo Clinic breaks it down even further by suggesting that "Mental illnesses, in general, are thought to be caused by a variety of genetic and environmental factors: Inherited traits. Mental illness is more common in people whose blood relatives also have a mental illness. Certain genes may increase your risk of developing a mental illness, and your life situation may trigger it.

Environmental exposures before birth. Exposure to environmental stressors, inflammatory conditions, toxins, alcohol or drugs while in the womb can sometimes be linked to mental illness. Brain chemistry. Neurotransmitters are naturally occurring brain chemicals that carry signals to other parts of your brain and body. When the neural networks involving these chemicals are impaired, the function of nerve receptors and nerve systems change, leading to depression."

Now far be it for me to attempt to argue with these experts especially since I do not possess their titles, status or degree of influence but as someone who suffers from a few listed mental illnesses, personal experience cause me to differ slightly. While I can wholeheartedly support Mayo Clinic's breakdown where it tells us that when it comes to inherited traits "certain genes may increase your risk of developing a mental illness and your life situation may trigger it", this would provide us some clue about a traumatic event bringing that illness to the forefront.

Good Genes or Bad Genes

Not saying that it is not but if the inherited trait part of Mayo Clinic's explanation is correct, then society may soon adopt a belief that this kind of gene can be detected and labelled so as to attempt to rid it from existence and keep those "bad genes" from causing any further harm to our society but in attempting to do would society then have to travel back in time to accomplish this goal.

What I mean is, if inherited then we must go as far back as Cain and Abel since this was the true beginning of man correct? I mean when Cain killed his brother Abel out of jealousy wasn't it then that this gene was planted in all of us? Could it be possible that even though there is no written record of Cain, and those who were around during those times, were ever labeled as having a mental illness, it was then that the seed was planted?

This would explain all of those Biblical fights written about in the Old Testament as well as all those wars and armed conflicts that followed. One section became jealous of another and decided to allow their bad gene to take control only to later find other means to justify the carnage and deaths. Could this explain why the infamous Billy The Kid shot a man for snoring after losing in a poker game or why after being welcomed to this New World by the Indians, we flipped to calling them savages and reducing them to reservations? Was this inherited trait buried deep inside those individuals and was allowed to rise to the surface to suit their agenda of taking instead of sharing?

This may be a lot to consider but one thing we know for sure. We know that life is a balance and with every ounce of bad there is an ounce of good. When it comes to a mental illness, each individual person must ask themselves whether we wish to exercise that good or bad gene. We know that it appears extremely more difficult to activate the good gene than it does to flip the switch on the bad one but that is also what separates us from other species which exist in this universe.

The choice of which you choose to unleash at any time in your existence is your’s and your’s alone. Control of which gene is activated is often dictated by what is happening at that particular time but even then individuals still remain the sole owner of that choice and proves with each passing hour, each passing day that mental illness is as common as the cold and it is time we stopped running from it.

There are so many different kinds of mental illness and each has its own causes and effects but one thing is sure, the type you may have does not make you broken, it does not make you defective, it does not make you worthless and it does not make you crazy. What it does make you is human and being human, we can choose whether we wish to be functional or non-functional. We can choose to own our illness or allow our illness to won us.

Introduction to the DSM and Just a Few Disorders

The following information is taken from the Diagnostic and Statistical Manual of Mental Disorders (DSM–5) for the express purpose of allowing all readers to get a sample of the many illnesses that are present within our society.

The American Psychiatric Association says the Diagnostic and Statistical Manual of Mental Disorders (DSM–5) is the product of more than 10 years of effort by hundreds of international experts in all aspects of mental health. Their dedication and hard work have yielded an authoritative volume that defines and classifies mental disorders in order to improve diagnoses, treatment, and research.

Autism spectrum disorder is characterized by persistent deficits in social interaction and communication in multiple life areas as well as restricted and repetitive patterns of behaviors. The DSM specifies that symptoms of autism spectrum disorder must be present during the early developmental period and that these symptoms must cause significant impairment in important areas of life including social and occupational functioning.

Attention-deficit hyperactivity disorder is characterized by a persistent pattern of hyperactivity-impulsivity and/or inattention that interferes with functioning and presents itself in two or more settings such as at home, work, school, and social situations. The DSM-5 specifies that several of the symptoms must have been present prior to the age of 12 and that these symptoms must have a negative impact on social, occupational, or academic functioning.

Bipolar disorder is characterized by shifts in mood as well as changes in activity and energy levels. The disorder often involves experiencing shifts between elevated moods and periods of depression. Such elevated moods can be pronounced and are referred to either as mania or hypomania.

Anxiety disorders are those that are characterized by excessive and persistent fear, worry, anxiety and related behavioral disturbances. Fear involves an emotional response to a threat, whether that threat is real or perceived. Anxiety involves the anticipation that a future threat may arise. Types of anxiety disorders include:

Panic disorder is a psychiatric disorder characterized by panic attacks that often seem to strike out of the blue and for no reason at all. Because of this, people with panic disorder often experience anxiety and preoccupation over the possibility of having another panic attack.

Separation anxiety disorder is a type of anxiety disorder involving an excessive amount of fear or anxiety related to being separated from attachment figures. People are often familiar with the idea of separation anxiety as it relates to young children's fear of being apart from their parents, but older children and adults can experience it as well. When symptoms become so severe that they interfere with normal functioning, the individual may be diagnosed with separation anxiety disorder.

Acute stress disorder, which is characterized by the emergence of severe anxiety within a one month period after exposure to a traumatic event such as natural disasters, war, accidents, and witnessing a death.

Adjustment disorders can occur as a response to a sudden change such as divorce, job loss, end of a close relationship, a move, or some other loss or disappointment. This type of psychological disorder can affect both children and adults and is characterized by symptoms such as anxiety, irritability, depressed mood, worry, anger, hopelessness, and feelings of isolation.

Post-traumatic stress disorder can develop after an individual has experienced a stressful life event. Symptoms of PTSD include episodes of reliving or re-experiencing the event, avoiding things that remind the individual about the event, feeling on edge, and having negative thoughts. Nightmares, flashbacks, bursts of anger, difficulty concentrating, exaggerated startle response, and difficulty remembering aspects of the event are just a few possible symptoms that people with PTSD might experience.

Dissociative disorders are psychological disorders that involve a dissociation or interruption in aspects of consciousness, including identity and memory.

Eating disorders are characterized by obsessive concerns with weight and disruptive eating patterns that negatively impact physical and mental health. Feeding and eating disorders that used to be diagnosed during infancy and childhood have been moved to this category in the DSM-5.

Narcolepsy is a condition in which people experience an irrepressible need to sleep. People with narcolepsy may experience a sudden loss of muscle tone.

Insomnia disorder involves being unable to get enough sleep to feel rested. While all people experience sleeping difficulties and interruptions at some point, insomnia is considered a disorder when it is accompanied by significant distress or impairment over time.

Restless legs syndrome is a neurological condition that involves having uncomfortable sensations in the legs and an irresistible urge to move the legs in order to relieve the sensations. People with this condition may feel tugging, creeping, burning, and crawling sensations in their legs resulting in an excessive movement which then interferes with sleep.

Kleptomania involves an inability to control the impulse to steal. People who have kleptomania will often steal things that they do not really need or that have no real monetary value. Those with this condition experience escalating tension prior to committing a theft and feel relief and gratification afterwards.

Pyromania involves a fascination with fire that results in acts of fire-starting that endanger the self and others.

Intermittent explosive disorder is characterized by brief outbursts of anger and violence that are out of proportion for the situation. People with this disorder may erupt into angry outbursts or violent actions in response to everyday annoyances or disappointments.

Conduct disorder is a condition diagnosed in children and adolescents under the age of 18 who regularly violate social norms and the rights of others. Children with this disorder display aggression toward people and animals, destroy property, steal and deceive, and violate other rules and laws. These behaviors result in significant problems in a child's academic, work, or social functioning.

Oppositional defiant disorder begins prior to the age of 18 and is characterized by defiance, irritability, anger, aggression, and vindictiveness. While all kids behave defiantly sometimes, kids with oppositional defiant disorder refuse to comply with adult requests almost all the time and engage in behaviors to deliberately annoy others.

Alcohol-related disorders involve the consumption of alcohol, the most widely used (and frequently overused) drug in the United States.

Cannabis-related disorders include symptoms such as using more than originally intended, feeling unable to stop using the drug, and continuing to use despite adverse effects in one's life.

Inhalant-use disorder involves inhaling fumes from things such as paints or solvents. As with other substance-related disorders, people with this condition experience cravings for the substance and find it difficult to control or stop engaging in the behavior.

Stimulant use disorder is a new category now found in the DSM-5 that involves the use of stimulants such as meth, amphetamines, and cocaine.

Tobacco use disorder is characterized by symptoms such as consuming more tobacco than intended, difficulty cutting back or quitting, cravings, and suffering adverse social consequences as a result of tobacco use.

Delirium, also known as acute confusional state, that develops over a short period of time (usually a few hours or a few days) and is characterized by disturbances in attention and awareness.

Antisocial personality disorder is characterized by a long-standing disregard for rules, social norms, and the rights of others. People with this disorder typically begin displaying symptoms during childhood, have difficulty feeling empathy for others, and lack remorse for their destructive behaviors.

Avoidant personality disorder involves severe social inhibition and sensitivity to rejection. Such feelings of insecurity lead to significant problems with the individual's daily life and functioning.

Borderline personality disorder is associated with symptoms including emotional instability, unstable and intense interpersonal relationships, unstable self-image, and impulsive behaviors.

The Forgotten Disorder

Of all the previously mentioned disorders that were present in the DSM-5 one that was not seen or maybe simply missed is abandonment. Abandonment often stems from childhood loss. This loss could be related to a traumatic event, such as the loss of a parent through death or divorce. It can also come from not getting enough physical or emotional care. These early childhood experiences can lead to a fear of being abandoned by others later in life. It may negatively affect any other relationships a person develops, whether they are intimate, social, or professional. Stress or overwhelm can contribute to emotional abandonment. People with unmet needs often have a difficult time meeting the needs of others. Some degree of abandonment fear can be normal. But when fear of abandonment is severe and frequent, it can cause trouble. It may impact how a person's relationships develop. People who felt abandoned as children may be more likely to repeat this pattern with their children."

This may go a very long way in explaining why many of us make huge mistakes when bringing a child into this world, not because it is our intention to pass along our bad gene but simply because we fail to understand more about what we are going through and how abandonment may have affected us starting as a child and now as an adult.

There are still times where I will second-guess myself or feel unworthy of something good that happens to me. My dad leaving the family to fend for themselves, has no doubt left me feeling like I have to work that much harder to even be accepted. His choice to leave left me thinking that if my own dad left me, why anyone else would stick around. Very little thought and credit was given to my mom for sticking around and raising me and my nine other siblings as best she could. I guess it goes back to that old saying that you always pine for that which you don't have and ignore the blessings that you do get.

Now that I have learned more about abandonment, I have seen myself become much better at handling this emotion but before then it is safe to say I was a complete mess. I feared that I would never amount to anything even though I was told and clearly shown different. If I was rejected for any reason, from being chosen to play a game with the other kids to not being picked to lead the class in prayer, it was enough to have me withdraw into my shell and barely speak another word for most of the remaining time I was in that environment.

When it came to relationships, it was just about the same. Every single relationship was short-lived and many of them ended quite badly, even when my partner was fully committed to me, I could not stay fully committed to her. The most frustrating part needed to feel loved and appreciated so badly, I still self-sabotaged relationships that ran past its normal course of one week. Because I had no clue why this was happening, it became my normal and only after learning more about abandonment and myself did it ever change to where I have much better control over it than in the past.

So for those who find themselves in a relationship where a child or children become a part of it, I ask that you do not allow that child to miss any opportunity to bond with, associate with or get to know the other biological half of who they are. The only exception, in my opinion, would be if their safety would be in jeopardy or the other parent has made it very clear that he/she truly does not want anything to do with the child.

The Connection

I am sure that by now, many of you have seen many of the same disorders appear in several different places. This is because, contrary to what some may want you to believe, these illnesses are connected. While it may begin as abandonment, it can swiftly convert or morph into a serious case of fears or anxiety. Sometimes they will follow closely behind the other and often times they may feel like that they have come together.

This is when life seems to become overwhelming and if we have not equipped ourselves with newer coping skills to deal with this, frustration and depression soon follows. For many this connection of illnesses seems unbreakable and often times they are but the ability of any one of us to deal with them properly is never outside of our grasp. We do it as we do many other things and make a conscious decision not to allow this illness to become a disorder.

We have witnessed a connection to how these illnesses can also lead to a physical degrading and if we are to be honest with ourselves, this physical degrading is often placed first on our to-do lists and we quickly seek medical attention for it. The funny thing is how we are so quick to seek medical attention for any physical ailment but we shrink away from seeking help for mental attention. It's like we are okay with sitting down at the kitchen table and helping our children with their homework but run and hide when it's time to help them with their mental work.

The American Psychiatric Association has a saying that "mental health is the foundation for emotions, thinking, communication, learning, resilience and self-esteem. Mental health is also key to relationships, personal and emotional well-being and contributing to community or society." This has never been truer than the lessons available here in this book. I can only add that I honestly believe that a strong mental health is the key to a stronger physical health, so while you are running back and forth getting medical help for your physical ailments, try getting some help for your mental ailments too. You might just come to realize that taking care of your mental health will eliminate the need to seek help for your physical health.

The only proof I can offer you for my suggestion above is to consider this. A trail for a new drug is happening and the group collected to do the trail is divided into two. The first group gets the real drug while the second group is made to believe that they got the real drug when in reality they did not. Check the numbers on those who did not get the real drug but feels just as good, if not better, than those who did get it. And by the way, check the number of those who got the real drug but believe so strongly that they did not even those conducting the study cannot convince them that they are feeling better. In the military we were told "mind over matter" and in this situation it truly is that.

The Only Cure is Coping Skills

I've found myself amazed at some who promise to cure your mental illness and right behind that amazement comes my anger at how it could be possible especially considering the trigger being a traumatic event. Think about it, the only way to cure it would be to develop a time machine, go back in time and prevent the event from ever happening or possibly getting a hold of that memory erasing pen used in the movie Men in Black.

While there is no cure for mental illness, there are coping skills to help you control them. To quote from the experts we call upon the website "Very Well Mind" whose article titled "40 Healthy Coping Skills for Dealing With Uncomfortable Emotions" which can be found at https://www.verywellmind.com/forty-healthy-coping-skills-4586742, they suggest that "there are two main types of coping skills: problem-based coping and emotion-based coping. Problem-based coping is helpful when you need to change your situation, perhaps by removing a stressful thing from your life. Emotion-based coping is helpful when you need to take care of your feelings when you either don't want to change your situation or when circumstances are out of your control." Which avenue you choose to take is strictly up to you to decide.

I personally believe that another ways to cope would be breathing because often times that split second before we explode with emotions are often spent not taking a breath and the second would be to redefine. What I mean by that is often what stresses us the most is how we perceive events and if we perceive a certain event in a negative manner then those bad genes begin to bubble. For example, if you are anything like me, you hate for someone to tell you what to do. What if instead of seeing as them telling you, you see it as them suggesting it? A suggestion is much less damaging to your character or ego than someone feeling as if they are in any position to tell you.

For those times you are the one attempting to convince another person of something, keep in mind that, like you, once they have made up their minds, a team of wild horses won't make them change it so why allow yourself to be frustrated. Inform them because you really need to inform them but expect nothing in return. Sometimes you may be surprised that when you just informed without expectations, what you desired to happen, may just happen.

Functional versus Non-Functional

Basically all that I am saying regardless of how we came about being exposed to contracting a mental illness, we got one now and the only two choices we have is to control it or allow it to control us. I, personally, refuse to let anything or anyone control me so we know which direction I choose to go in. The question is which door you will choose. Asking for help is a true sign of a hero because a hero is never afraid to ask for help if needed. You can either take my word for it or consider that even Superman had Super Friends.

No one is saying that it won't be hard and no one saying that everything will turn out peachy everytime but to not do anything is not only extremely foolish but very dangerous considering those bad genes just waiting to explode all over people. Imagine the fall out if family is involved, or your children. Stacking one thing on top of another might be a good idea in the beginning but if not watched and attended to, it will turn into a really big mess.

Redefine it like this, for so long you have went out of your way to take care of others, I am now asking you to go out of your way and now take care of you. To say that you are not worthy or that you do not deserve to enjoy your life tells me that you have never looked into a mirror. It's time to stop trying to be everything others want you to be and be true to who you are. If you are still working to try and find out who you are then great because self-discovery is a gratifying feeling as you do it. There is a saying that if you spend all your time being who others wants you to be, who will spend that time being you?

Redefine that individual, even if it's you, who are under some grand illusion that their way is the one and only way because as they continue this narcissistic path with this ludacris idea of "one size fits all" they will be the ones who miss out on the glory and splendor that is learning more

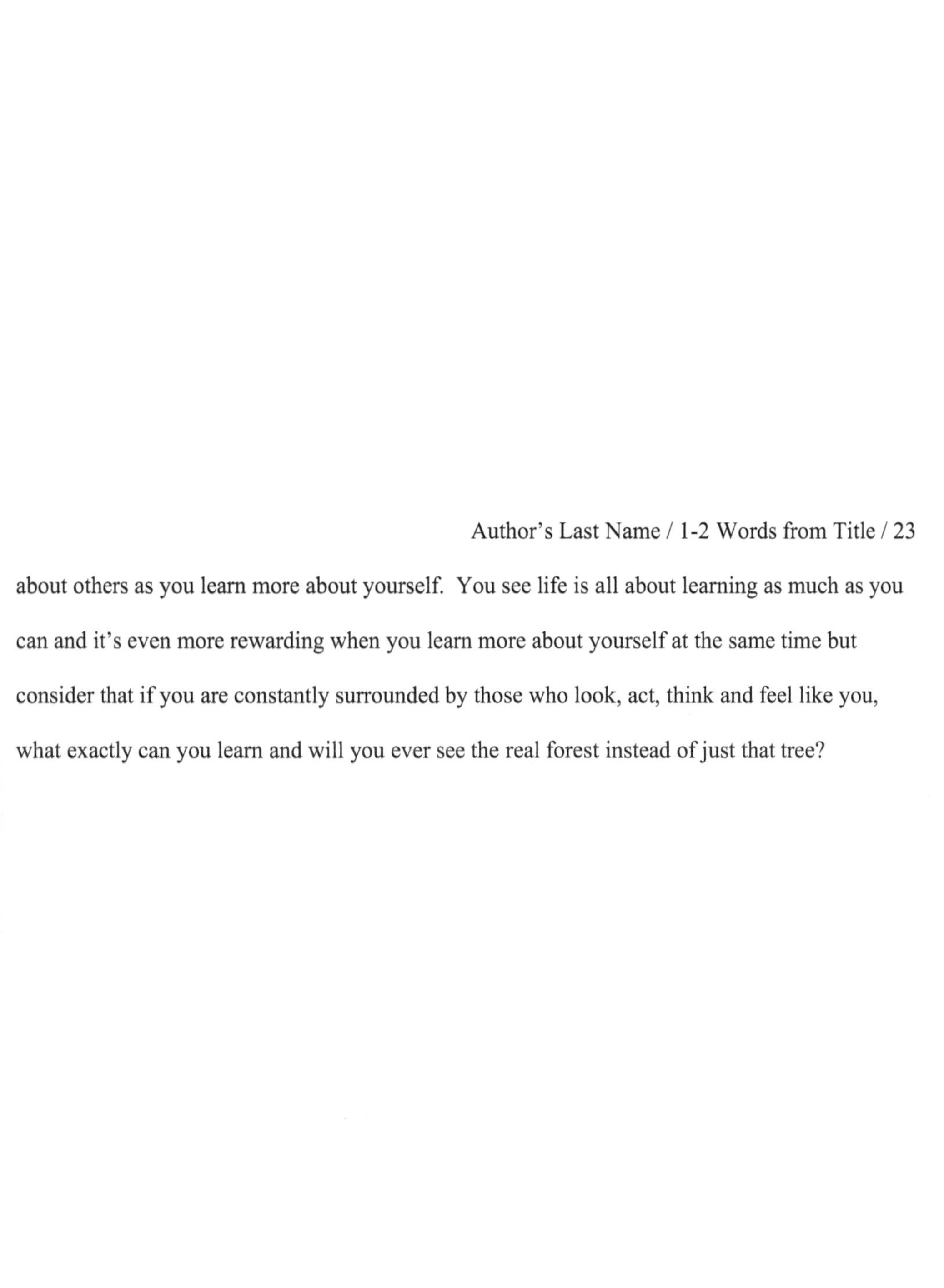

about others as you learn more about yourself. You see life is all about learning as much as you can and it's even more rewarding when you learn more about yourself at the same time but consider that if you are constantly surrounded by those who look, act, think and feel like you, what exactly can you learn and will you ever see the real forest instead of just that tree?

RonSue's Tree of Mental Illness

It is my hope and desire that this book helps you to see mental illness in a completely different light that it is not about being defective, broken or crazy. Dealing with a mental illness does not mean that you are worthless, less-than, alone and unloved. What dealing with a mental illness truly means is the courage of one to own it before it owns them and the strength of character and spirit never to allow anyone or anything to convince them otherwise. Mental illness is as common as the cold and as previously stated, like a cold can and often will turn into something more devastating if it goes untreated and undiagnosed. It does not take a rocket scientist to know that you are not quite yourself on some days and no one should ever feel as they have to shoulder all that alone. Simply put, again, even Superman had Super Friends.

This final subject speaks on the tree of mental illness and this reality was developed simply to try and help you better understand mental illness and why it is nothing to be afraid or ashamed of. It is my belief that the primary cause of something is the answer that we all seek when we feel that something just isn't right. The failure to figure it out or get the answers needed to understand what is happening to us individually, leads to many other things and sometimes to very unwise decisions.

I believe that the root cause of all mental illnesses is the illness of abandonment. I see it as the root of this tree because in our early years we form the purest example of unconditional love, from your first psychological bond with birth parents to that first childhood crush and with that comes the enormous expectation that what we are told by those we love is gospel. So when a parent promises to always love us and never go away, yet years later die or divorce and move away, we have a very hard time reconciling that. We often times seek answers to why and when those answers do not come for whatever reason, we then form our own answers and often times it are that we must have done something to drive them away. Failure to hear from that person or the people we carry this love for, continues to add to our slowly shrinking feeling of self-worth and the longer we go without an explanation, the more frustrated we become.

This frustration is the base of the tree along with displacement. Now we are easily frustrated by almost anything and anyone, not really because of what they did to us, even though if asked we will find a reason to say it is, but since we do not know for sure why those loved ones left, we are left with guessing. We also become quickly frustrated with strangers and eventually settle with the feeling that if our own parents did not wish to be around us then who else will. We tend to then develop this need for self-protection and even if a relationship is going well, find a way to sabotage it ourselves just for the sake of saving us the pain to falling too deep for that person who will ultimately leave us. Displacement now replaces rational thinking and we soon began to find all types of reasons to blame others for our lack of character ethics or morals because the weight of carrying around this idea that those we loved unconditionally left.

Our decision not to seek help with this, leads directly to our illness becoming a disorder which takes over every aspect of our lives and makes all of our decisions for us. When that happens, you have just crossed over from having a mental illness to now having a mental disorder and that dynamic is where the other branches of this tree spring from. One branch may be depression, the other anxiety; another may be dependent while another may be bipolar. There can be many branches of this tree and they all can exist in common with each other or independently.

Regardless, to gain a much better handle and control over any mental illness, you must first seek out and discover the root. Once you have accepted and begin dealing with that root, can only then will you be able to easily grab a hold of all those branches and wipe them into shape. Society sees the answer to mental illness in ranges of medication and dosage but I strongly disagree. Mental illness is about mental process of events and occurrences in your life and as long as you can place your own label on these things when they happen, the more functional you shall remain. There is one other thing that I need you to know before I go and that is regardless of what happens in your earthly life, know that God will always love you and that each of us have a special job to do that only we can do. No need to attempt suicide, when you have completed the job God has sent you here to do, he will call you home. I also need you to know that it is true that what doesn't break you will make you stronger and dealing with a mental illness can make you the strongest that you have ever been or ever thought you could be. The desire to better yourself for those you love and those who love you will make you begin to see that perfection is not about having no imperfections but moreover how you adapt, overcome and conquer those imperfection to make you the most perfect imperfect person that you can be.

About The Author

Ronnie (Ron) Manns was born in Ripley Tennessee on July 7, 1962, but hails from Brownsville, Tennessee. He enlisted in the United States Marine Corps in September 1980 and departed for Marine Corps Basic Training right after graduating Haywood High School. Upon graduating Basic Training out of Parris Island, South Carolina and obtaining his chosen Military Occupational Skill as a Military Policeman and made stops in Camp Pendleton, California; Okinawa, Japan; Camp Lejeune, North Carolina and Yuma, Arizona. He served during the conflicts of Beruit, Grenada, Panama, and Desert Storm. He was honorably discharged in April 1991 and now resides in Arizona. Ron is a proud dad of two biological sons Cordney Brandon Manns and Terren Lee Manns as well as his three biological daughters Terra Lynn Manns, Apryl D. Harper, Ashley D Harper and his adopted daughter Shanequa Lashawn Kent-Manns. Ron is also helped to raise his niece and nephews Katisha Moton, Jermarque Taylor-Manns and Deondre Moton as foster children. He is blessed to have by his side his lovely wife and longtime friend, Susan M. Manns. He currently holds the title of Certified Crisis Intervention Counselor and Behavioral Health Professional after mastering each of the 7 modules necessary to obtain those titles along with achieving over 3,600 hours of direct contact with patients defined as suicidal.

www.ingramcontent.com/pod-product-compliance
Lightning Source LLC
Chambersburg PA
CBHW031430230726
48656CB00020B/2346

* 9 7 8 1 0 9 6 6 6 8 1 9 0 *